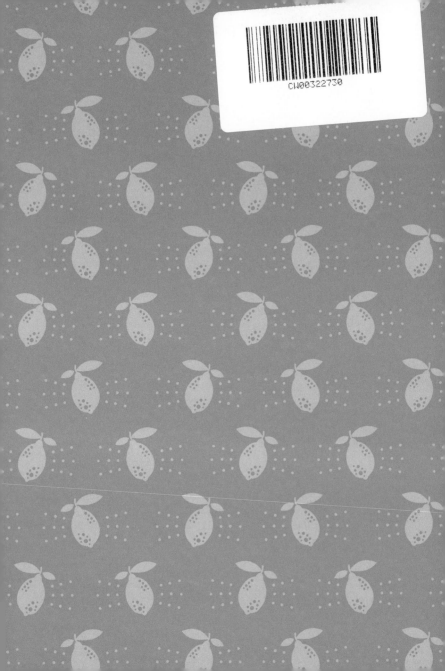

LEMONS
are a
GIRL'S BEST
FRIEND

First published in Great Britain in 2017 by Modern Books
An imprint of Elwin Street Productions Limited
14 Clerkenwell Green
London EC1R 0DP
www.modern-books.com

All recipes serve one unless otherwise specified.

ISBN 978-1906761-93-6

10 9 8 7 6 5 4 3 2 1

Printed in China

LEMONS
are a
GIRL'S BEST
FRIEND

Janet Hayward

Illustrations by Jonwen Jones

m

CONTENTS

HONEY 64

Raw Salad with Honey
Honey and Peppermint
  Lip Balm

LEMONS 68

Lemon and Parsley Lentil Salad
Lemon and Honey Face Mask

OATS 72

Bircher Muesli
Oat and Lavender Bath Soak

PINEAPPLES 76

Tropical Pineapple and Coconut
Pineapple Foot Scrub

AVOCADOS 80

Green Breakfast Smoothie
Avocado Hair Treatment

COCONUTS 84

Green Coconut and Mango
  Cream
Coconut Oil and Lavender Body
  Cream

CUCUMBERS 88

Cucumber and Mint Raita
Cooling Face and Body Mist

FENNEL 92

Fennel, Orange and Mint Salad
Fennel Seed Eye Comfort

GREEN TEA 96

Green Tea with Mint and Ginger
Green Tea Steam Facial Treatment

MINT 100

Zingy Minty Salad
Refreshing Mint Hair Rinse

BLACK GRAPES 104

Black Grape and Ricotta Salad
Black Grape Toner

BLUEBERRIES 108

Blueberry and Oat Cookies
Blueberry Exfoliator

CHIA SEEDS 112

Chia Breakfast Smoothie
Chia Skin and Lip Oil

DATES 116

Date and Beetroot Bliss Balls
Date, Yoghurt and Honey
  Face Mask

OLIVES 120

Marinated Olives with Feta
Olive Oil Hair Treatment

SEAWEED 124

Nori Wraps
Seaweed Face Mask

RECIPE FINDER 128

INTRODUCTION

What's not to love about lemons? Rich in vitamin C, perfect for cleansing and brightening, and with the power to restore your body's pH balance, lemons are packed full of powerful nutrients that not only offer multiple health benefits, but can also boost your natural beauty from within.

It isn't only lemons – there is a whole spectrum of 'superfruits' and 'superveggies' with the power to give you an enviable, radiant glow that even the most expensive beauty products can't create. The secret lies in the naturally intense colours of the superfoods, as the strong pigments not only make them look appealing, but are also extremely beneficial flavonoid compounds that have powerful antioxidant and anti-inflammatory effects on our bodies. Antioxidants help to neutralize free radicals that can cause damage and inflammation to healthy cells – including skin, hair and nails. So the more brightly coloured fruit and vegetables in your diet, the stronger your immune system and general health will be. These same ingredients can also work wonders when prepared and applied to your skin and body as personalized, natural beauty treatments.

For each season nature provides us with colourful and nutrient-dense foods that we need to keep us feeling healthy and looking amazing at that time of year. This book guides you through the best fruits and vegetables to choose and how to turn them into delicious recipes and pampering beauty treatments that will ensure you look and feel like a glamazon all year round!

CHERRIES

Crisp, juicy cherries are at their best during the summer
months. Mainly grown in the temperate climates of Europe and
North America, these fleshy stone fruits feature in a wide range
of delicious recipes both sweet and savoury.

The cherry's beautiful, deep-red colour comes from a powerful
antioxidant, anthocyanin, which acts as an anti-inflammatory and
helps keep the entire body fit and healthy. Cherries are particularly
rich in the minerals potassium, magnesium and iron, as well as the
B vitamins folic acid, niacin and riboflavin. Vitamins A and C
are present, too. Assisting in collagen production, these useful
nutrients help maintain the elasticity of the skin, keeping
it looking young and fresh.

This superfruit also contains sleep-regulating melatonin,
which could suggest that cherries can contribute to a good night's rest.
What could be a better boost for all-round beauty than that?

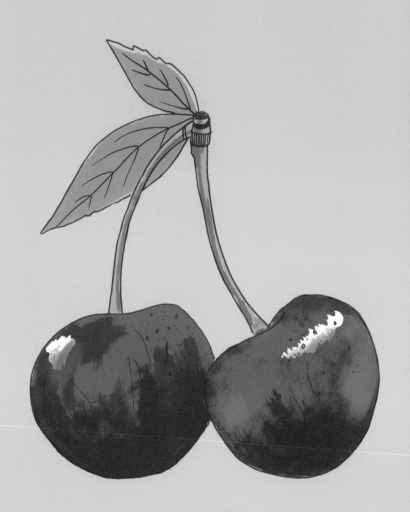

SOUR CHERRY AND MINT GRANITA

Inside: Enjoy this antioxidant- and vitamin-rich refresher to enliven your complexion.

You will need:

450g fresh cherries • 3 tablespoons coconut sugar • 6 fresh mint leaves, plus extra for garnish • 250ml water

To prepare:

Remove the stones from the cherries and purée in a blender with the coconut sugar, six mint leaves and water – the mix can be smooth or chunky, depending on your preference.

Spread the purée evenly over a shallow baking tray and freeze for forty-five minutes, until solid. Return to the blender for a short blast to form the granita. Spoon into serving glasses and top each with a fresh mint leaf. Serve immediately.

CHERRY LIP TINT

Outside: Hydrate and moisturize your lips
with this pretty tinted balm.

You will need:

6 ripe, deep-red cherries • 1 tablespoon coconut oil • 1 vitamin
E capsule • small glass pot with lid

To prepare:

Halve the cherries, remove the stones and place the flesh in a
small glass bowl. Add the coconut oil and the contents of the
vitamin E capsule. Place the glass bowl over a small saucepan
of boiling water to melt the ingredients and release the juice
from the cherries. Once happy with the colour of the mixture,
remove the cherry halves. Allow the mix to cool before
pouring into the small glass pot and storing in the fridge.

To use:

Apply this cherry-red tint to your lips for a hint of natural
moisturizing colour.

CRANBERRIES

Native to North America and Canada, cranberries generally grow from spring through to winter, and need a large amount of sunlight to ripen fully. Their benefits can be enjoyed all year round, however, in the guise of dried cranberries and juice.

This zesty superfruit's tartness is an instant indication of the natural acidity that makes the cranberry such a great all-round health food. The lush, red berries contain antioxidants, including proanthocyanidins, which can offer protection from tooth decay and inflammatory conditions. They are also a good source of vitamins A and C, the essential B vitamins, and the minerals potassium and manganese – a perfect cocktail for healthy skin, hair and nails.

Bursting with phytonutrients, in juice form cranberries are often recommended for treating urinary tract infections. This is because the juice makes urine acidic, meaning bacteria are less likely to linger and flourish in the bladder.

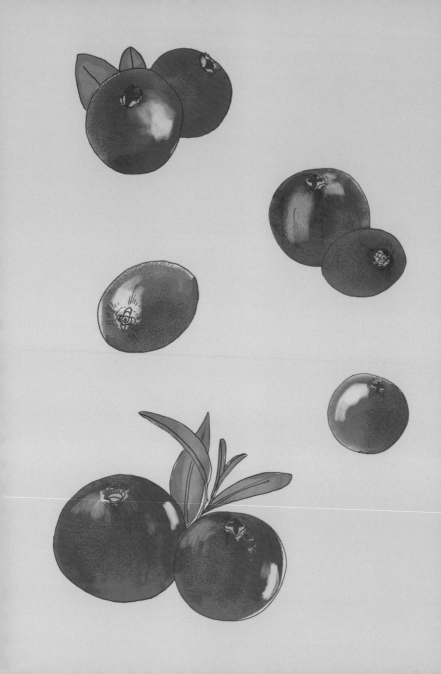

CRANBERRY-POACHED PEAR

Inside: Calm your whole body with this
light, zesty palate cleanser.

You will need:

1 ripe pear • 100ml cranberry juice • 1 teaspoon honey
• ½ cinnamon stick • Greek yoghurt (optional)

To prepare:

Peel the pear, cut into halves and remove the core. Place in a
small saucepan with the cranberry juice, honey and cinnamon
stick. Cover and simmer over a low heat for ten minutes.
Remove the lid and simmer for a further five minutes to
reduce the cranberry sauce some more.

Serve the poached pear with a spoonful of the cranberry
sauce and a spoonful of Greek yoghurt, if desired.

CRANBERRY AND ROSEHIP TONING WATER

Outside: Enjoy a smoother, softer face
after using this skin-toning water.

You will need:

3 tablespoons unsweetened cranberry juice • 3 tablespoons
witch hazel • 3 drops rosehip oil • small glass bottle with
screw top

To prepare:

Carefully decant the cranberry juice, witch hazel and rosehip
oil into the glass bottle and shake vigorously to blend.

To use:

After cleansing, pour a little of the toning water onto a
dampened cotton pad and wipe gently across your face to
remove any residual make-up and dead skin cells.

GOJI BERRIES

Goji berries are native to Tibet, China and the Himalayas, where they have been used for thousands of years for their medicinal benefits. Also known as wolfberries, these plump little superfruits boost immunity, help to increase alertness and improve circulation. Autumn is the season for fresh goji berries, although they can be hard to find in the West. Thankfully, they are available in dried form all year round, so you need never go short!

Loaded with antioxidants and boasting high levels of vitamin C, goji berries are unique in that they contain all the essential amino acids and a high concentration of protein to keep the body healthy and youthful-looking. These tiny, bitter-sweet fruits have no fewer than 21 trace minerals, including a very high level of iron, as well as selenium and zinc.

Be in no doubt, adding a teaspoon of goji berries to your breakfast cereal or a dessert will ensure a glowingly healthy mind, body and spirit!

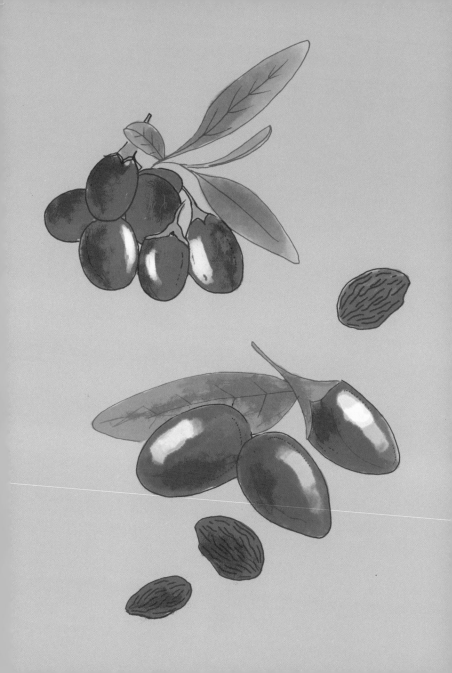

GOJI POWER SMOOTHIE

Inside: Say goodbye to mid-morning snacks with this filling, high-protein breakfast smoothie.

You will need:

1 banana • 1 kiwi fruit • 3 tablespoons dried goji berries

• 1 tablespoon cacao powder • 250ml coconut water

• 3 tablespoons yoghurt

To prepare:

Peel and chop the banana and kiwi. Place in a blender and add the goji berries, cacao powder, coconut water and yoghurt. Blend together until smooth.

GOJI BERRY EXFOLIATOR

Outside: Apply this nourishing exfoliator for smooth, supple and youthful-looking skin.

You will need:

1 tablespoon dried goji berries • ½ avocado

To prepare:

Roughly chop the goji berries and blend with the avocado to make a paste.

To use:

Gently massage onto your face and neck to exfoliate, moisturize and enliven the skin.

POMEGRANATES

Originating in the Middle East, the Mediterranean and northern India, the pomegranate has long played a prominent role in the history, art and culinary traditions of those regions. With bright, ruby-red juice packed into tiny seeds, this superfruit is as visually attractive as it is healthy. At its best, its flavour is a unique blend of sweet and sour, and the jewel-like seeds shine in recipes both sweet and savoury.

Flourishing in autumn, pomegranates bring amazing health and beauty benefits just in time for the winter months ahead. Known for their powerful anti-ageing and anti-inflammatory properties, these red-skinned fruits are rich in potassium, vitamin C, polyphenols and vitamin B6. These combine to fight free-radical damage. They also boost collagen production, so promoting springy, youthful-looking skin.

Drink pomegranate juice to give your immune system a boost – a glass of the richly coloured nectar offers twice the antioxidant power of the same volume of red wine or green tea.

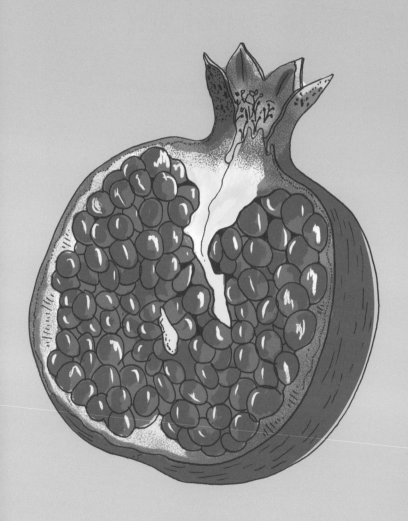

HALLOUMI, ORANGE AND POMEGRANATE SALAD

Inside: Help combat free-radical damage with this fresh, antioxidant-rich salad.

You will need:

250g halloumi • 2 oranges • 1 pomegranate • ½ bunch of fresh basil • olive oil • juice of ½ lemon • sea salt • black pepper

To prepare:

Cut the halloumi into eight equal slices and grill until golden. Cut away the skin of both oranges and divide into segments, taking care to remove the pith. Arrange the halloumi slices and orange segments on a serving platter.

Remove the seeds from the pomegranate, sprinkle them over the halloumi and orange and top with torn basil leaves. Lightly dress the salad with olive oil and lemon juice, adding sea salt and black pepper to taste.

POMEGRANATE AND COCONUT FACIAL TREAT

Outside: Refresh and hydrate your skin with this highly nourishing, anti-ageing treatment.

You will need:

2 tablespoons pomegranate seeds • 1 tablespoon coconut oil
• 1 tablespoon honey

To prepare:

Combine all the ingredients in a bowl, distributing the juice from the pomegranate seeds evenly throughout the mixture.

To use:

Gently massage the mixture onto your face to loosen dry skin cells. Leave it in place for five minutes to hydrate and moisturize. Rinse the mixture off using warm water and gently pat your skin dry with a clean, soft towel. It will feel soft and smooth with a radiant glow.

STRAWBERRIES

Juicy, sweet and reaching their peak at the height of summer, strawberries are highly alkalizing. They are packed full of fibre and vitamins – including vitamin C – and contain high levels of antioxidants, all of which helps to guard against disease and inflammation. This great-tasting and popular superfruit also aids digestion and is renowned for helping to regulate blood sugar levels.

These bright, potent fruits are rich in anthocyanins, manganese and potassium, which help to protect the heart and regulate blood pressure. Perhaps this could explain why the strawberry is considered an aphrodisiac! The combination of powerful nutrients – such as magnesium with vitamin A – helps to promote optimum skin health for a naturally radiant glow.

If you are looking for the perfect smile, look no further. Crushed strawberries mixed with a little salt provide a great natural way to whiten teeth while sweetening the breath at the same time.

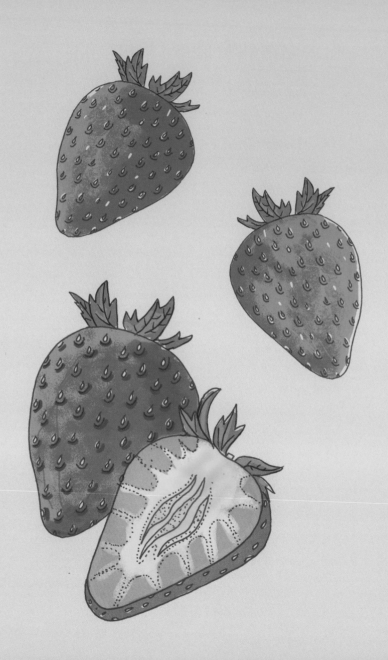

STRAWBERRY, FENNEL AND GOAT'S CHEESE SALAD

Inside: Combine these two superfoods in the perfect salad for an alkaline diet.

You will need:

450g strawberries • 1 large fennel bulb • 1 cucumber • 1 small goat's cheese • 4 tablespoons olive oil • 2 tablespoons white wine vinegar • 2 teaspoons Dijon mustard • 1 teaspoon honey • sea salt • black pepper

To prepare:

Wash the strawberries, remove their hulls and slice. Wash the fennel bulb, trim the fronds remove the core and finely slice. Wash the cucumber, then peel and slice finely. Combine the three ingredients in a large serving bowl. Cut the goat's cheese into small pieces and dot over the salad.

In a separate bowl, combine the olive oil, white wine vinegar, Dijon mustard and honey. Add sea salt and pepper to taste. Pour this dressing over the salad and serve immediately.

GENTLE STRAWBERRY
FACIAL EXFOLIANT

Outside: Apply this enzyme-action exfoliator
for smooth and supple skin.

You will need:

75g strawberries • 1 tablespoon milk • 1 tablespoon jojoba oil

To prepare:

Mash the strawberries in a small glass bowl and mix together
with the milk and the jojoba oil.

To use:

Gently apply the exfoliant all over your face, taking care to
avoid the eyes. Leave on for five minutes (eight minutes if
you have oily skin) and rinse with warm water. Pat dry gently,
then apply your usual serum or moisturizer.

TOMATOES

Globe, plum, cherry – there are several thousand varieties of this smooth-skinned superfood. Although most commonly served in salads or as a topping for Italian staples such as pasta and pizza, the tomato is actually a fruit that originated in Central America. Traditionally a summer ingredient, today the tomato tastes delicious all year round, which is great news for health and beauty.

These plump, red gems are particularly rich in lycopene, a unique and powerful antioxidant compound that helps to protect cells from free-radical damage. Lycopene is also effective in offering the skin some protection from ultraviolet (UV) rays. Tomatoes also contain high levels of potassium – a vital component of body cells and fluids – alongside calcium, iron and manganese.

Effective levels of vitamin A and beta-carotene help to keep skin healthy and contribute to good vision, while vitamin C maintains the smooth functioning of the immune system.

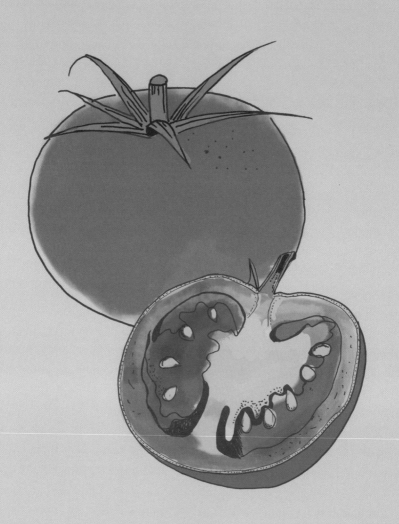

TOMATO AND BASIL BRUSCHETTA

Inside: Give your immune system a boost
with this easy lunch.

You will need:

2 teaspoons truffle oil • 2 thick-cut slices sourdough or spelt
bread • 2 ripe tomatoes • ½ avocado • pinch dried chilli flakes
• 2 fresh basil leaves • sea salt • black pepper

To prepare:

Drizzle one teaspoon of truffle oil equally across the two slices
of bread. Roughly chop the tomatoes and place in a small
bowl. Cube the avocado and add it to the bowl with the dried
chilli flakes, salt and black pepper to taste, and the remaining
truffle oil. Gently combine and allow the flavours to mingle.

Spoon the mixture onto the slices of bread and top each with a
fresh basil leaf, cut into strips.

TOMATO FACE MASK

Outside: Treat acne-prone or oily skin
with this deep-cleansing mask.

You will need:

2 ripe tomatoes • 1 tablespoon honey

To prepare:

Cut the tomatoes in half and scoop out the pulp and seeds into
a small bowl. Using a fork, mash the tomato to a smooth paste,
add the honey and combine thoroughly.

To use:

Smooth the paste over your face, taking care to avoid the
eyes and lips. Leave on for ten minutes, then use a tissue to
remove. Rinse the skin with warm water and pat dry. A mild
tingling sensation is usual after applying the mask, but if it
persists or is uncomfortable, remove it.

CHAMOMILE

Delicate German chamomile belongs to the summer-flowering daisy
family and is popular as a soothing tea, best enjoyed at bedtime.
Used throughout history in medicine and as a beauty treatment, this
herb's calming effect can help relieve anxiety and depression, while
giving the immune system a boost at the same time.

Consumed as a tea, chamomile can benefit those suffering from nausea,
tummy upsets and menstrual cramps, and can reduce colic in babies.
This is because the herb increases levels of the amino acid glycine in the
body, which enables muscle relaxation. A good source of antioxidants
that can help regulate blood sugar, chamomile also contains traces of
vitamin A and folate, as well as calcium, magnesium and potassium.

Applied to the body, chamomile can soothe sensitive skin and help
ease sore, red patches associated with eczema, dermatitis, acne,
and even sore scalps. An extra bonus for blondes is that the
herb can also be used as a final rinse for fair hair, lifting the
colour for a sun-kissed effect.

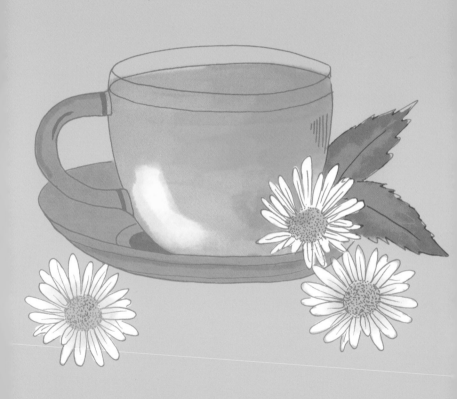

CHAMOMILE AND LEMON SPRITZ

Inside: Team calming chamomile with lemon for
a refreshing alkalizer for your body.

You will need:

250ml freshly boiled water • 5 chamomile tea bags
• 2 teaspoons raw honey • 1 lemon • sparkling water

To prepare:

Pour the boiling water over the chamomile tea bags and leave
them to infuse for five minutes to make a concentrated liquid.
Add the honey and stir to melt, then add the grated zest and
juice of the lemon.

Pour the tea into a tall glass jug and add sparkling water to
taste. Serve over ice for a refreshing and relaxing summer
drink, garnished with a slice of lemon.

SLEEPY-TIME CHAMOMILE BATH SALTS

Outside: Soothe sensitive skin with this
relaxing bathtime treat.

You will need:

250g Epsom salts • 4 chamomile tea bags or 2 tablespoons
chamomile flowers tied in a muslin cloth

To prepare:

Place the Epsom salts and the chamomile tea bags in the
bottom of the bath and run the hot water until they are fully
covered. Allow the chamomile to infuse into the bathwater for
ten minutes, before running more water to produce the
perfect temperature for a relaxing bath.

To use:

For the maximum benefit, leave the tea bags or cloth in the
water as you relax in the bath before bedtime. This will help
promote a restful beauty sleep.

PEACHES

A delicious and aromatic stone fruit that reaches its peak at the height of summer, the peach was first cultivated in China and is now enjoyed across the globe. Sun-blushed and velvet-skinned, the juicy inner flesh of this superfruit can be yellow with a distinctive zesty flavour, or white with a sweeter tang.

Both yellow and white peaches are a great source of antioxidants, vitamins, minerals and dietary fibre, making them an all-round superfood when promoting optimum health. Rich in immune-boosting antioxidants, including beta-carotene, which gives them their pretty orange colour, peaches are especially beneficial in maintaining healthy, glowing skin. They are an excellent source of vitamin A to promote flawless skin texture and vitamin C to assist in collagen production that keeps complexions youthful. Essential minerals include potassium, magnesium and selenium to ensure healthy cells throughout the body.

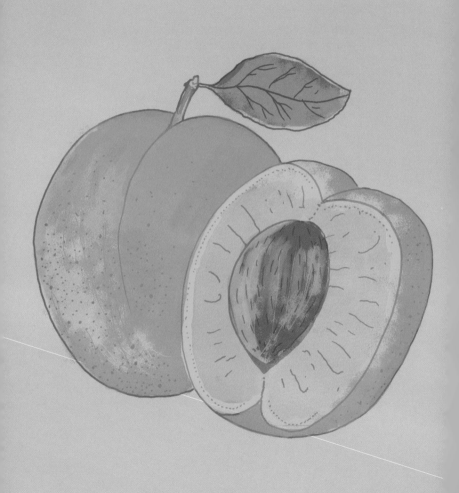

PEACH, TOMATO AND MOZZARELLA SALAD

Inside: Invigorate skin with this antioxidant- and vitamin-rich salad.

You will need:

2 ripe peaches • 3 medium heirloom tomatoes • 1 mozzarella ball • 5 basil leaves • 1 tablespoon olive oil • 1 teaspoon Dijon mustard • sea salt • black pepper

To prepare:

Halve and stone the peaches then cut into small chunks and place into a serving bowl. Cut the tomatoes into quarters and chop the mozzarella ball into small pieces then add to the bowl. Mix together the olive oil, Dijon mustard and salt and pepper to taste then pour the dressing over all the ingredients in the bowl. Add the basil leaves and gently combine to create a delicious healthy salad.

GENTLE PEACH EXFOLIATING MASK

Outside: Use this vitamin A-rich exfoliating mask
to encourage cell turnover.

You will need:

1 ripe peach • 1 tablespoon honey • 2 tablespoons oats

To prepare:

Peel and halve the peach. Discard the stone and mash the
fruit into a puree in a small glass bowl. Add the honey and the
oats and combine to form a thick paste.

To use:

Smooth the mixture over your face taking care to avoid the
eye area. Leave on for fifteen minutes then massage gently to
remove loosened skin cells. Rinse your face with warm water
and pat dry with a clean, soft towel to leave glowing, refreshed
skin ready for your serum or moisturizer.

CINNAMON

Harvested from the bark of a tree native to Sri Lanka, cinnamon is a highly powerful antioxidant. Thanks to its distinctive aroma and delicious, almost sweet, flavour, this spice features in many recipes for warming baked goods and is frequently associated with winter. That's a good thing too, since this woody superfood harbours naturally effective antimicrobial properties that make it a great support to the body's immune system during the cold and flu season.

Cinnamon is also a great source of manganese – essential for the healthy functioning of the metabolism and the nervous system, as well as the formation of connective tissues, healthy bones and regulation of blood sugar levels. Mixing a teaspoon of cinnamon with raw honey can help soothe sore throats or ease respiratory problems, while some find the scent of cinnamon helps boost concentration and brain activity!

The health and beauty benefits of this superspice can be enjoyed throughout the year by adding a light sprinkling to cereal and yoghurt or as a finishing touch to a cup of coffee or hot chocolate.

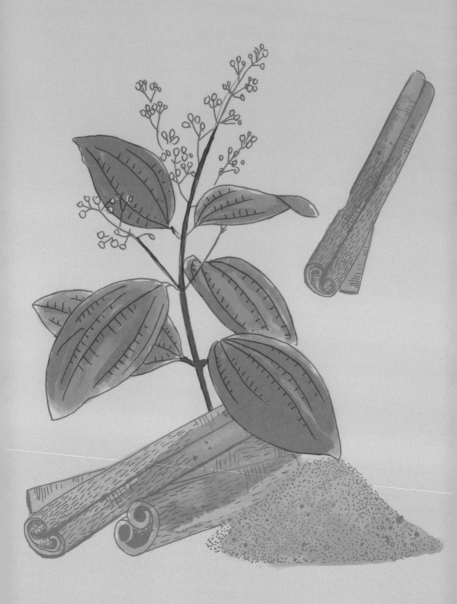

CINNAMON AND GINGER MELON

Inside: Enjoy the calming effects of this refreshing fruity concoction.

You will need:

½ cantaloupe melon • ½ honeydew melon • 1cm piece fresh ginger • 250ml water • 1 cinnamon stick • 1 teaspoon ground cinnamon • 100g rapadura (or coconut sugar if unavailable) • juice of ½ lemon • Greek yoghurt

To prepare:

Cut both melons into equal-sized cubes and place in a serving bowl. Peel and chop the ginger finely and place in a small saucepan with the water, cinnamon stick, ground cinnamon, rapadura and lemon juice.

Heat until the rapadura has melted, then simmer over a low heat until the mixture has reduced and thickened to a light syrup. Pour over the melon cubes and decorate with the cinnamon stick. Serve with Greek yoghurt.

CINNAMON SPOT TREATMENT

Outside: Reduce the redness of sore spots with this deep-clean treatment.

You will need:

1 tablespoon honey • ½ teaspoon ground cinnamon

• cotton buds

To prepare:

Combine the honey and cinnamon together to form a thick, smooth paste.

To use:

Use a cotton bud to dab a generous amount of the paste onto the spot. Leave for ten minutes then rinse away. Repeat morning and evening.

MANGOES

Delicious, nutritious and the ultimate symbol of summer, the mango is a real feel-good fruit. Commended for aiding concentration, weight loss and digestion, it also restores elasticity and hydration for youthful-looking skin and lusciously healthy hair. Mangoes are literally packed with vitamins and minerals that regulate, cleanse and nourish the body. They contain high levels of probiotic fibre, making this smooth-skinned superfruit a healthy, tummy-friendly snack or dessert.

A mango's high levels of alkaline-balancing tartaric and malic acids, as well as powerful vitamins A and C, help boost the immune system and keep eyes clear and healthy. B vitamins are great for balancing hormones and keeping the heart healthy, while rich sources of iron, calcium, beta-carotene, potassium, magnesium and copper help keep blood, skin and hair in tip-top condition.

Although naturally sweet when ripe, mangoes have a low glycaemic index (41–60) so you won't experience the 'sugar-rush' of a chocolate bar after eating. Nevertheless, you will feel full, satisfied and blessed with healthy energy.

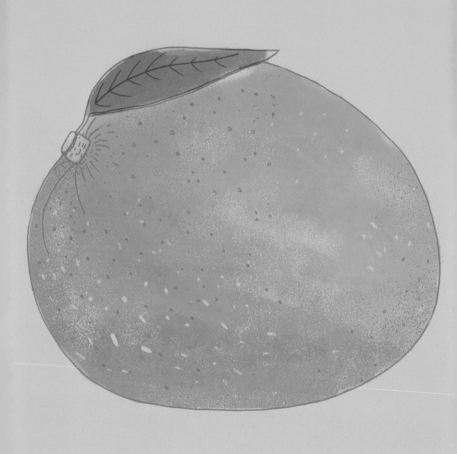

MANGO SALSA

Inside: Eat this fiery, probiotic
salsa to aid digestion.

You will need:

2 ripe mangoes • 1 small red onion • 1 small red chilli
• 1 tablespoon extra-virgin olive oil • juice of ½ lime • small
bunch of fresh coriander leaves • sea salt • black pepper

To prepare:

Peel and pit the mangoes and slice into strips. Finely chop the
red onion and the chilli, taking care to remove the chilli seeds.
Place all together in a small serving bowl and add the olive oil
and the lime juice.

Top with torn coriander leaves and mix together, adding salt
and pepper to taste. Cover and leave in the fridge for half an
hour to allow the flavours to combine before serving.

MANGO AND AVOCADO CLEANSER

Outside: Enrich your skin with this nourishing cocktail of vitamins and good oils.

You will need:

1 ripe mango • ½ ripe avocado • 1 tablespoon natural yoghurt

To prepare:

Place the flesh of the mango and the avocado in a small dish and add the yoghurt. Mash, and mix to a smooth consistency.

To use:

Gently massage the cleanser into your face, neck and décolletage for three minutes. Rinse with warm water and pat dry before applying your usual serum or moisturizer. For a deeper cleanse, keep the face mask on for ten minutes before rinsing.

PAPAYAS

At its best in early summer, a ripe papaya, with its juicy, bright-orange flesh, is delicious simply with a squeeze of lime. It also combines well with other fruits or vegetables to make a delicious low-calorie smoothie or dessert – ideal for those bikini days ahead!

Green, or unripe, papaya is popular in savoury, Asian-style dishes and contains high levels of papain, an enzyme that naturally tenderizes meat. This tropical superfruit also contains high levels of phytonutrients, minerals and vitamins, as well as soluble dietary fibre, which aids digestion. With a higher vitamin C content than even a lemon, the papaya is a great immune booster.

Potent levels of vitamin A, beta-carotene and lutein combine with essential B-complex vitamins, potassium and calcium to make the papaya a powerful antioxidant that will keep you in the very best of health, from your hair right down to your toenails.

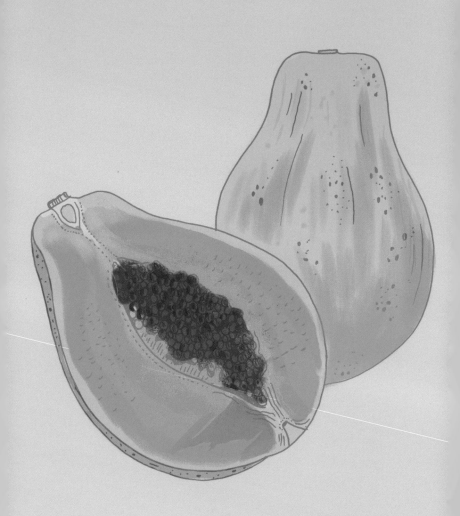

PAPAYA, AVOCADO AND CUCUMBER SALAD

Inside: Combine this trio of superfoods for glossy hair and glowing skin.

You will need:

1 ripe papaya • 1 ripe avocado • ½ cucumber • small bunch of fresh mint • 1 tablespoon olive oil • juice of ½ lemon • sea salt • black pepper

To prepare:

Peel the papaya, remove the seeds and cut the flesh into slices. Repeat with the avocado and place both in a serving bowl. Add the cucumber, cut into chunks, and top with torn mint leaves. Prepare the dressing by mixing the olive oil and lemon juice with salt and pepper to taste.

Pour the dressing over the salad and toss gently before serving. This salad pairs well with roast chicken.

HONEY AND PAPAYA TREATMENT
FOR HANDS AND FEET

Outside: Smooth rough or dry skin with
this enzyme-rich mix.

You will need:

½ ripe papaya • 3 tablespoons honey • 1 tablespoon rolled oats

To prepare:

Scoop out the flesh of the papaya into a small glass bowl and add the honey and the oats. Combine thoroughly.

To use:

Soak your hands and feet in warm water for five minutes and then coat in the papaya mixture. Leave for thirty minutes before massaging the mixture gently into your skin. Rinse in warm water to remove.

SWEET POTATOES

Native to Central and South America, the sweet potato was introduced to Europe by Christopher Columbus towards the end of the fifteenth century. It was not long before its popularity spread across the rest of the globe. Although most of us see orange when we think of this starchy tuber, purple varieties grow, too.

Orange or purple, this supervegetable is rich in manganese, copper, essential B vitamins, potassium, phosphorus and fibre. It also contains choline – a nutrient that helps maintain cell membranes and the transmission of cell impulses. Consequently, it assists with muscle movement, memory and sleep. Sweet potatoes are high in the phytonutrient beta-carotene, which the body converts to vitamin A, and in anti-inflammatory anthocyanins. Combined with slow-release carbohydrates, this is all good news for blood sugar regulation.

Cook this root vegetable in its skin with a small amount of fat. That way you'll get the maximum benefits from all it has to offer.

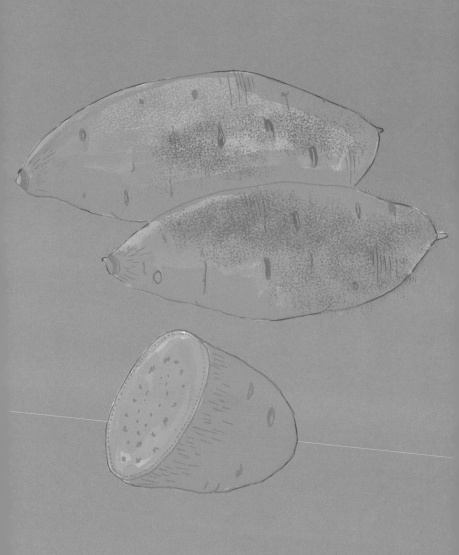

SCRUMPTIOUS SWEET POTATO SMASH

Inside: Top up your beta-carotene levels for a boost of anti-inflammatory vitamin A.

You will need:

2 sweet potatoes • 1 tablespoon ghee or olive oil • 2 tablespoons grated Parmesan cheese • sea salt • black pepper

To prepare:

Scrub the sweet potatoes and cut them into small cubes, leaving the peel on. Boil in hot water until the flesh is soft, then strain. Add the ghee or olive oil and mash the cubes lightly with a fork. Add salt and pepper to taste.

Transfer the mash to an ovenproof serving dish, top with the grated Parmesan cheese and grill until golden brown. Serve immediately with fish or chicken.

SWEET POTATO DÉCOLLETAGE RUB

Outside: Exfoliate and moisturize with this hydrating skin treatment.

You will need:

1 sweet potato • 1 tablespoon yoghurt • 1 tablespoon coconut oil

To prepare:

Peel and cube the sweet potato and boil until soft. Add the yoghurt and coconut oil and combine thoroughly using a stick mixer to make a paste.

To use:

Smooth the paste over your décolletage and neck. Leave for fifteen minutes to exfoliate, hydrate and nourish this delicate area. You can also use this treatment all over your face, taking care to avoid the eye area.

ALMONDS

Nutrient dense and with a high (good) fat content, a handful of almonds makes the perfect beauty snack.

An excellent source of vitamin E, B vitamins, potassium, calcium, magnesium, phosphorus and iron, as well as essential mono- and polyunsaturated fatty acids, the almond is a powerhouse of goodness that will literally make skin and hair glow and encourage strong nails. These sweet, milky kernels are also rich in antioxidants, which help keep the whole body healthy – even the heart.

Enjoy almonds raw or dry-roasted – or soak them overnight before adding to breakfast cereal (this makes the nutrients more easily digestible). A truly versatile superfood, the almond's benefits can also be found in a glass of almond milk, in almond butter or in biscuits made with almond meal.

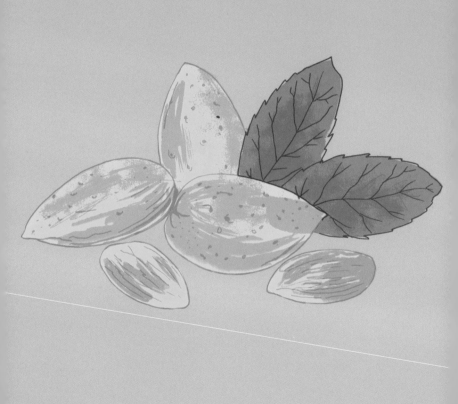

ALMOND BREAKFAST SMOOTHIE

Inside: Give your skin a healthy glow with this
magnesium- and vitamin E-rich smoothie.

You will need:

250ml almond milk • 1 banana • 125g frozen raspberries

• 1 tablespoon almond butter • 1 teaspoon honey

• 1 tablespoon rolled oats (optional) • ground cinnamon

To prepare:

Place all the ingredients except the cinnamon in a blender and
blitz together to make a thick and creamy smoothie. Dust the
top with cinnamon and serve immediately.

SWEET ALMOND OIL FACIAL CLEANSER

Outside: Apply this nutty treatment for smooth, supple and hydrated skin.

You will need:

4 tablespoons sweet almond oil • 2 tablespoons coconut oil
• small clean glass jar with a lid • cotton cloth square

To prepare:

Pour the two oils into the glass jar, screw on the lid and shake to combine thoroughly. Store in the fridge.

To use:

Gently warm the oil between your fingertips before massaging all over your face to loosen make-up and grime. Rinse a cotton cloth in warm water and then gently wipe across your face to remove the cleansing oil and surface grime. Rinse the cloth thoroughly and leave to air dry.

CIDER VINEGAR

Cider vinegar has been credited with amazing health benefits for centuries. It is made by crushing apples and then adding yeast to ferment the natural sugars. A bacteria is introduced, which turns the liquid into acetic acid. Small quantities of proteins, enzymes and healthy bacteria then form, which are believed to give this tangy superfood its antioxidant, antibacterial and antimicrobial qualities.

A great balancing act, cider vinegar is helpful in restoring healthy bacteria in the stomach, resulting in better digestion and higher energy levels. At the same time, it can help regulate blood sugar and cholesterol levels. Mixed with honey and lemon juice, cider vinegar is a useful antioxidant-rich treatment for colds during winter months, killing bacteria and soothing sore throats. Used externally, it is an ideal all-natural cleaning fluid!

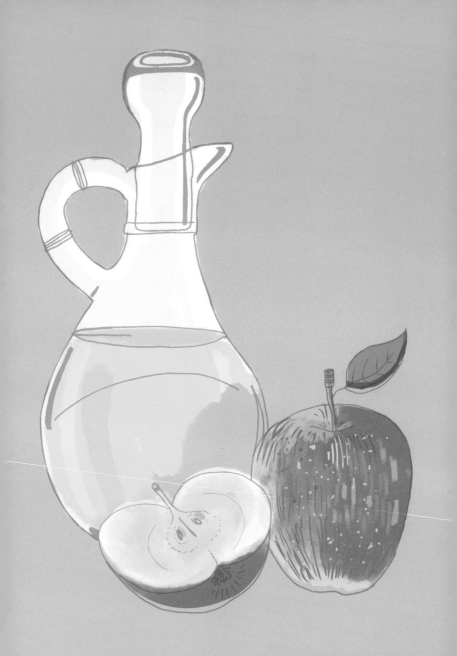

CIDER VINEGAR MARY

Inside: Mix this tastebud-tingling tomato juice to ease digestion.

You will need:

250ml fresh tomato juice • 2 tablespoons cider vinegar
• 1 splash Worcestershire sauce • sea salt • black pepper
• celery stalk

To prepare:

Pour the tomato juice into a tall glass and add the cider vinegar and Worcestershire sauce. Sprinkle with salt and pepper to taste. Stir with the celery stalk before serving.

SUPER SCALP CLEANSE

Outside: Soothe a flaky scalp with this naturally antimicrobial, enzyme-action rinse.

You will need:

250ml cider vinegar • 250ml water • 2 drops lavender oil

To prepare:

Mix the cider vinegar and the water together, then add the lavender oil and stir to mix.

To use:

To treat an itchy, flaky scalp, gently massage the mixture into your scalp. Leave for twenty minutes to allow the cider vinegar to alter the pH balance, then rinse and shampoo and condition as usual. For the ultimate hair shine treatment, use the mixture in the final rinse when washing your hair.

HONEY

A product of the bee's hard labour, honey plays a vital role in the ecology of the planet. It also happens to be a golden elixir that has been used for centuries as a delicious superfood and a highly effective medicine. Powerful antioxidant, antibacterial and antimicrobial benefits bring an impressive boost to the immune system while protecting against ageing and infection – even when applied topically.

With high levels of fructose and glucose, both of which are easily absorbed by the body, honey gives an instant energy boost. B-complex vitamins are also present, alongside calcium, copper, iron, magnesium, manganese, phosphorus, potassium, sodium and zinc. Important amino acids help maintain and repair the body's connective tissues.

Depending on the climate and environment of the bees, some types of honey have more powerful effects than others. For example, Manuka honey, made by bees that flock to the manuka bush in New Zealand, has particularly effective antimicrobial properties.

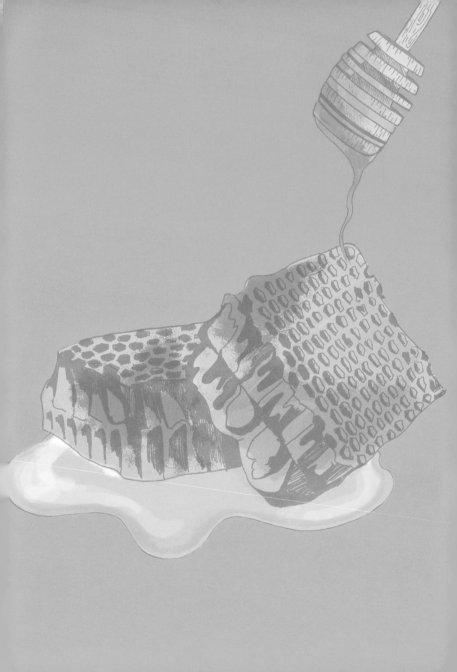

RAW SALAD WITH HONEY

Inside: Give your immune system a boost with
this nutrient-rich, honey-flavoured dressing.

You will need:

¼ white cabbage • 1 carrot • 1 green apple • 1 tablespoon cider
vinegar • 1 tablespoon olive oil • 2 teaspoons honey • juice of ¼
lemon • chilli flakes • sea salt • black pepper

To prepare:

Shred the white cabbage finely and place in a serving dish.
Scrub the carrot, wash the apple and slice both into fine sticks,
then add to the dish.

Pour the cider vinegar, olive oil, honey and lemon juice into a
small glass bowl and add the chilli flakes. Whisk together until
thoroughly combined. Add salt and pepper to taste, before
pouring the dressing over the serving dish. Stir well to coat
the ingredients fully.

HONEY AND PEPPERMINT LIP BALM

Outside: Keep your lips hydrated in winter with this antibacterial lip treat.

You will need:

1 tablespoon coconut oil • 1 teaspoon honey • 2 drops peppermint oil • small glass storage pot with lid

To prepare:

Spoon the coconut oil and honey into a small glass bowl and heat over a saucepan of hot water until thoroughly melted and combined. Remove from the heat.

Once the mixture has cooled, add the peppermint oil and stir thoroughly. Pour into the storage pot and allow to cool and firm up before screwing on the lid.

To use:

Apply the tingly lip balm to your lips for soothing hydration.

LEMONS

With their powerful immune-boosting, antioxidant, antibacterial and antiviral properties, lemons have amazing natural healing properties that offer great health and beauty benefits inside and out. Although lemons taste acidic, they are actually alkaline, which means they help to regulate the body to an ideal balance of pH 7.30–7.45. Lemon juice also aids digestion and helps cleanse the liver. This all adds up to a healthier body, which means clearer skin and shinier hair!

But it doesn't stop there. The mighty lemon offers 88 percent of your daily dose of vitamin C – renowned for fighting colds and flu bugs – along with potassium and magnesium, both of which help promote healthy skin. For double the impact, lemons can be used in a number of beauty treatments to cleanse, refresh and add a youthful glow: skin looks more radiant, hair looks shinier, nails look whiter with a little help from the humble lemon. One easy way to include lemon in your daily routine is to squeeze the juice of half a lemon into a glass of room temperature water, then sip first thing in the morning.

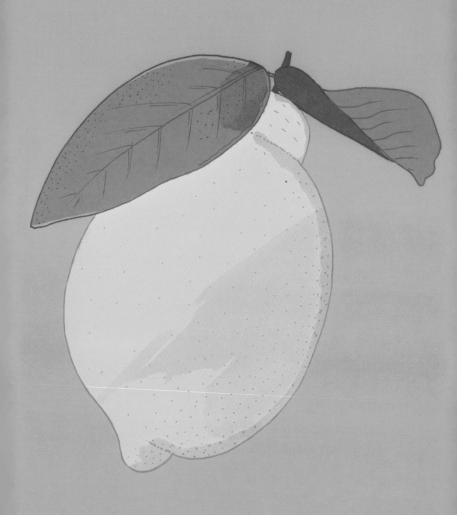

LEMON AND PARSLEY LENTIL SALAD

Inside: Eat this refreshing, alkalizing and cleansing
salad for an all-over body glow.

You will need:

1 red pepper • 1 cucumber • 1 small red onion • 190g cooked
brown lentils • small bunch of fresh parsley • juice of 1 lemon
• 2 teaspoons Dijon mustard • ¼ teaspoon salt • black pepper
• 80ml extra-virgin olive oil

To prepare:

Chop the red pepper, the cucumber and the red onion and
place in a large bowl. Add the cooked lentils. Chop the parsley
and place in a blender with the lemon juice, mustard, salt and
pepper, then gradually add the olive oil to create the dressing.

Pour the dressing into the bowl and carefully mix all the
ingredients together. Serve with a grilled chicken breast or
a poached salmon fillet.

LEMON AND HONEY FACE MASK

Outside: Revive dry skin with this exfoliating, soothing and moisturizing treat.

You will need:

4 tablespoons lemon juice • 4 tablespoons honey

• 4 tablespoons almond oil

To prepare:

Mix together the lemon juice, honey and almond oil in a small bowl.

To use:

Apply the mask to your face, taking care to avoid the eye area. Leave for fifteen minutes, then rinse off with warm water and pat dry. Your skin will feel soft, smooth and moisturized. To help brighten areas of skin pigmentation or acne scars, add an extra tablespoon of lemon juice and reduce the quantity of almond oil.

OATS

Traditionally a favourite winter breakfast, oats are a supergrain containing important nutrients that help maintain a healthy body and glowing skin. They are a great source of both soluble and non-soluble dietary fibre. Beta-glucan is a soluble fibre that can lower cholesterol and regulate blood sugar levels; while the non-soluble fibre in oats helps to keep the digestive system healthy.

Phytoestrogen helps to keep hormones balanced, while a high carbohydrate and protein content, along with essential fatty acids and important B complex vitamins and vitamin E, contribute to optimize health and energy.

Oats also contain a good level of calcium, manganese, zinc, selenium, copper, iron and magnesium – essential for the smooth functioning and repair of the body, including skin, hair and nails – making them an all-round great beauty superfood.

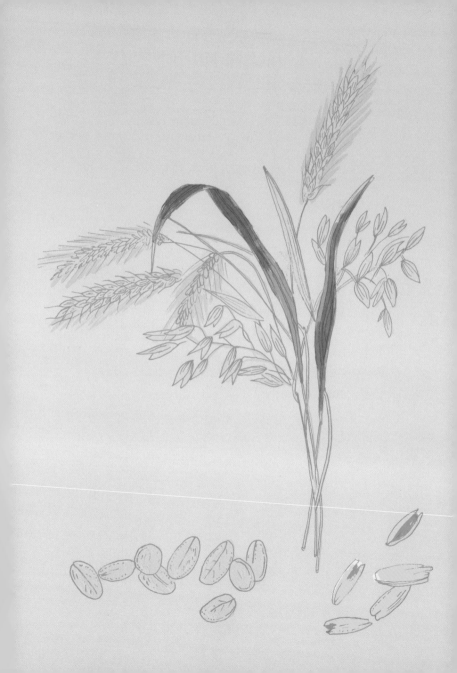

BIRCHER MUESLI

Inside: Calm your digestive system
with this oaty breakfast.

You will need:

90g rolled oats • 1 apple • 2 pitted dates • 1 tablespoon roasted
chopped hazelnuts • 1 tablespoon dried goji berries
• 2–3 tablespoons yoghurt

To prepare:

Place the oats in a bowl, add just enough water to cover and
soak overnight. Grate the apple, chop the dates and add to the
soaked oats along with the chopped hazelnuts and goji berries.
Add enough yoghurt to bind all the ingredients – plus a little
extra to taste.

OAT AND LAVENDER BATH SOAK

Outside: Restore health to your skin with this soothing bath time treat.

You will need:

45g rolled oats • 2 tablespoons milk powder • 4 drops lavender oil • muslin cloth • string

To prepare:

In a small bowl, combine the rolled oats with the milk powder and add the lavender oil. Spoon into the centre of the muslin cloth then gather the edges and tie with the string.

To use:

Place the bag in a running bath and leave to soak, like a tea bag, as you bathe. It will leave your skin feeling soothed and smooth. You will also feel relaxed and ready to enjoy a good night's sleep.

PINEAPPLES

A potent symbol of tropical goodness, the pineapple is fresh tasting
and simply packed with low-calorie goodness. Its zesty sharpness
comes from the presence of the enzyme bromelain, which helps
maintain a healthy digestive system by breaking down protein in food.
Consequently the pineapple is a great natural detox food and, thanks
to a high fibre content, is also beneficial for weight loss.

An excellent source of vitamin C and other cell-protecting
antioxidants, pineapples not only help collagen production
for healthy skin, but also provide a helpful boost to the immune
system, making them a great choice in winter.

Pineapple is also known for its high level of manganese –
a mineral that is essential in energy production – and thiamine,
which promotes healthy bones. Copper and potassium assist
with the production of red blood cells, so contributing
to healthy heart function.

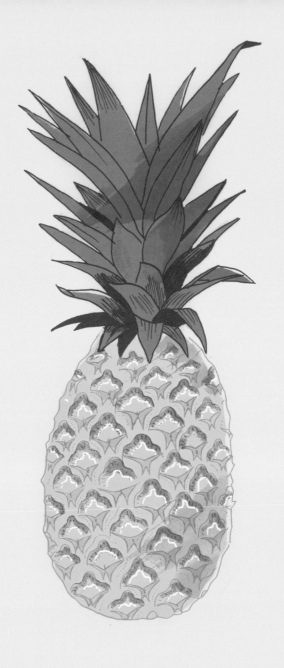

TROPICAL PINEAPPLE AND COCONUT

Inside: Top up your fibre intake with this
seemingly decadent dessert.

You will need:

$^1/_3$ pineapple • 45g muscovado sugar • 125ml coconut milk

• mint leaves, to serve

To prepare:

Peel the pineapple and cut into thick rings, then quarter
the rings. Place on a baking sheet and sprinkle with
muscovado sugar. Place under a hot grill for three to five
minutes, until brown. Remove from the grill and serve drizzled
with coconut milk and mint leaves.

PINEAPPLE FOOT SCRUB

Outside: Smooth feet and polish toenails
with this enzyme-acting scrub.

You will need:

2 tablespoons coconut oil • 330g fresh pineapple chunks

• plastic wrap • foot file

To prepare:

Heat the coconut oil and blend or mash together with the
pineapple chunks to make a mask.

To use:

Smooth the mask over your feet and cover with plastic
wrap to form socks. Leave for fifteen minutes to allow the
pineapple enzymes to soften any hard skin. Meanwhile, the
coconut oil will condition your feet. Remove the plastic wrap,
rinse your feet in warm water and gently file to remove
dead skin. Your feet will feel baby soft and smooth!

AVOCADOS

Healthy fats are important for the body to function at its best and eating half an avocado will provide 18g of very beneficial monounsaturated fat. In addition to helping disperse fat-soluble vitamins E and K around the body, monounsaturated fat is vital in maintaining the moisture levels in skin that keep it feeling soft and looking evenly toned and healthy. Hair feels softer and more silky and nails are more resilient. Vitamin E in avocados helps protect skin from visible signs of ageing, while vitamin C assists in the creation of elastin and collagen to keep skin looking youthful.

Avocados contain folate and potassium, vital for maintaining the nervous system and a healthy heart. Like all superfoods, they offer valuable anti-inflammatory and antioxidant protection. Simply adding a little of this superfruit to your salad or to a daily smoothie can make a world of difference to your general health and appearance. Enjoy a long season of this king of fruits from spring to autumn.

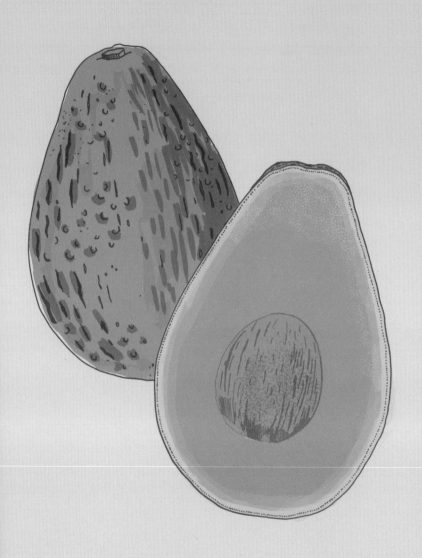

GREEN BREAKFAST SMOOTHIE

Inside: Drink this rich-tasting smoothie to give your body an alkaline boost.

You will need:

½ ripe avocado • 1 ripe banana • 1 kiwi fruit • 1 handful chopped kale • 310ml milk (dairy, soy or rice) • ¼ teaspoon cinnamon • 1 teaspoon honey (to taste)

To prepare:

Place all the ingredients in a blender and blast until smooth. Pour into a glass and serve immediately.

AVOCADO HAIR TREATMENT

Outside: Bring your split ends under control
with this tropical-smelling blend.

You will need:

2 tablespoons coconut oil • ½ avocado

To prepare:

Melt one tablespoon of the coconut oil in a small bowl placed
over a small saucepan of boiling water. Remove the bowl from
the saucepan and add the avocado, mashing to combine until
very smooth.

To use:

Before shampooing your hair, warm the remaining coconut oil
until clear and gently massage it into your scalp and roots. Comb
the avocado mixture through to the ends of your hair. Leave on
for ten minutes, then rinse with warm water before shampooing.

Try this treatment once a month to hydrate and condition hair.

COCONUTS

This tropical superfruit is loaded with vitamins — predominantly C and B — plus minerals and is high in antioxidant, anti-ageing compounds with anti-inflammatory, antibacterial and antiviral benefits for all areas of the body. When young, coconuts have an outer green husk and softer, more creamy 'meat'. As they mature, they develop a brown husk and the meat is much firmer. Green coconut 'meat' is rich in calcium and important fatty acids, while coconut oil has great antioxidant power that is retained even when heated during cooking.

Although green and mature coconuts both contain coconut water, the level of beneficial nutrients is much higher in the green coconut. With good levels of iron, calcium, manganese, magnesium, copper and phosphorus and impressively rich in potassium, green coconut water is ideal for restoring electrolyte levels during hot weather. It is also hugely hydrating, which is great news for skin and muscles. The water also makes an effective treatment for stomach upsets and can help regulate blood sugar levels.

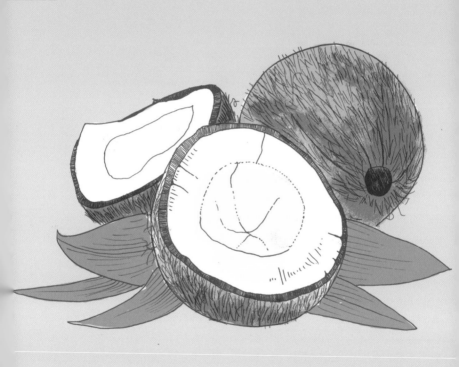

GREEN COCONUT AND MANGO CREAM

Inside: Give your immune system a boost with this delicious cream, rich in vitamins A and C.

You will need:

1 green coconut • 1 ripe mango • 1 teaspoon raw honey (optional)

To prepare:

Remove the top of the green coconut using a sharp knife. Pour out the coconut water and save for later. Use a spoon to scoop out the coconut meat and place in a blender. Slice the mango either side of the pit and scoop out the flesh. Add to the coconut in the blender and blend thoroughly, adding a little of the coconut water, until it forms a rich cream. Add the honey to taste if required.

Serve the cream as a topping for blueberries, strawberries or raspberries or enjoy on its own with toasted, flaked almonds.

COCONUT OIL AND LAVENDER BODY CREAM

Outside: Nourish all skin, even sensitive types, with this super-hydrating ointment.

You will need:

250ml coconut oil • 4 drops lavender oil • glass storage jar with lid

To prepare:

Spoon the coconut oil into a glass bowl and place over a saucepan of boiling water to melt the oil. Add the lavender oil and combine thoroughly, then remove from the heat.

Allow to cool and firm up, until almost solid. Then, using a hand mixer or a manual whisk, beat the mixture until it becomes light and creamy. Spoon into the jar and seal until ready to use.

To use:

Smooth the mixture over dry skin to moisturize and help you relax before bedtime.

CUCUMBERS

A popular ingredient in summer salads, cucumbers are rich in nutrients and contain two of the essential elements for healthy digestion: water and fibre. Approximately 96 per cent water, this refreshing superfood is a great cleanser, helping to flush out toxins that can dull the skin and hair. High levels of the minerals magnesium, potassium and silicon help restore a healthy, youthful glow to the skin and bring a glossy sheen to the hair. Vitamins A and C provide an immune boost that results in a natural radiance, while vitamin K ensures healthy capillaries and a strong nervous system.

Cucumbers can also have a calming effect: significant levels of vitamins B1, B5 and B7 are important for relieving anxiety and the effects of stress, while potassium helps reduce blood pressure and protects the heart. So there is some truth to the phrase 'cool as a cucumber' – both inside and out, as it happens, since everyone knows that a slice of cucumber is the best way to cool and soothe a sore eye.

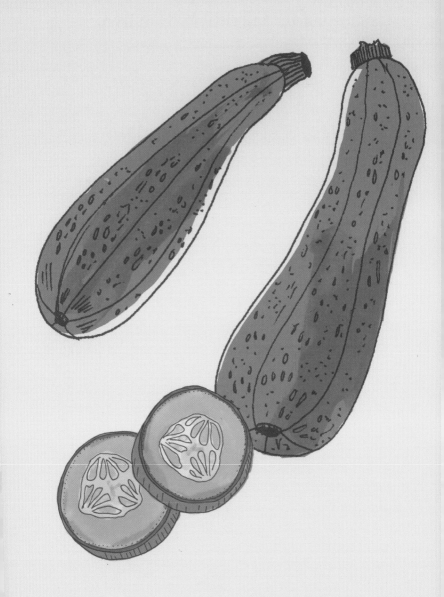

CUCUMBER AND MINT RAITA

Inside: Eat this cleansing side dish for
glowing skin and shiny hair.

You will need:

260g natural yoghurt • 1 tablespoon freshly chopped mint
• juice of ½ lime • 1 teaspoon cumin • 1 cucumber • sea salt
• black pepper

To prepare:

Stir the yoghurt, mint, lime juice and cumin together in a
small glass bowl. Finely chop the cucumber, leaving the skin
on, and add to the yoghurt mix with sea salt and black pepper
to taste. The raita is delicious served as a salad dressing or is
perfect with curries or spicy food.

COOLING FACE AND BODY MIST

Outside: Hydrate both face and body with this
refreshing, mineral-rich mist.

You will need:

2 cucumbers • 80ml rose water • cotton muslin cloth
• 100ml capacity spray bottle

To prepare:

Wash the cucumbers and finely grate them into a glass bowl.
Squeeze through the muslin cloth into a second glass bowl to
extract the cucumber water. Combine with the rose water,
then pour into the spray bottle.

To use:

Spray over the face and body to condition and cool throughout
the hot summer months. Stored in the fridge,this mist will last
for seven days.

FENNEL

With their delicate aniseed flavour, fennel bulbs are popular in salads and as a cooked vegetable in Mediterranean cuisine. Harvested during the winter months, fennel has many health benefits including helping with digestive problems, which is vital in making sure that your body gets the maximum health and beauty benefits from the superfoods you eat.

Fennel contains folic acid, which is essential for healthy cell development, as well as significant levels of antioxidant vitamin C – so important for a healthy immune system. The vegetable also has potassium for regulating blood pressure and keeping cells and fluids at their optimum functionality. Small quantities of trace minerals iron, calcium, magnesium, manganese, zinc, copper and selenium help to bring out the best in skin, hair and nails.

Finally, fennel's essential oil is often used in toothpaste and mouthwash for its antibacterial and antifungal properties.

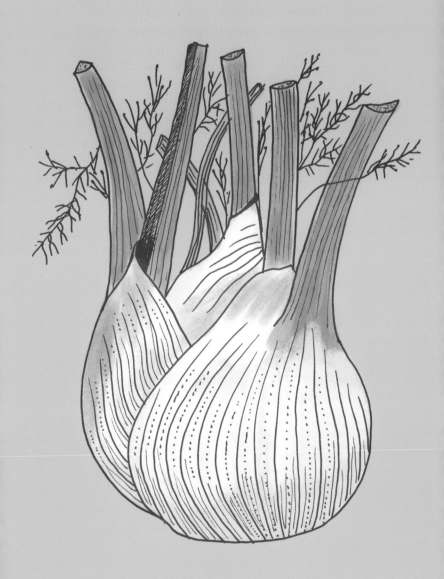

FENNEL, ORANGE AND MINT SALAD

Inside: Give your skin, hair and nails a welcome boost with this mineral-rich salad.

You will need:

1 bulb fennel • 1 navel orange • 1 tablespoon olive oil • juice of ¼ lemon • sea salt • black pepper • small bunch of fresh mint

To prepare:

Trim the fennel bulb, cut into wafer-thin slices and arrange on a serving plate. Using a sharp knife, peel the orange and cut into segments, removing the pith. Arrange the orange segments over the fennel slices and squeeze over any additional juice from the pith.

Mix the olive oil and lemon juice together and add salt and pepper to taste. Pour the dressing over the salad. Chop the mint leaves and sprinkle over the salad before serving.

FENNEL SEED EYE COMFORT

Outside: Reduce puffiness or redness to leave
your eyes looking clear and bright.

You will need:

250ml water • 2 teaspoons fennel seeds • cotton pads

To prepare:

Boil the water and pour over the fennel seeds. Leave to infuse
for five minutes, before straining the seeds and allowing the
eyewash to cool.

To use:

Soak two cotton pads in the fennel eyewash and place over
closed eyes for ten minutes.

GREEN TEA

Recognized as one of the healthiest drinks available, green tea contains a range of important nutrients to ensure a healthy mind, body and soul!

This refreshing elixir is rich in polyphenols, which have a powerful antioxidant and anti-inflammatory effect on the body, so protecting cells and molecules from free-radical damage. The drink also contains small quantities of amino acids and minerals that help to keep the body functioning well and can even help lower cholesterol levels and maintain a healthy metabolic rate.

Flavonoids called catechins can help to slow down bacteria and virus growth, making green tea a great choice in winter time. Surprisingly, for a healthy drink, this superfood also contains caffeine. Often considered a negative property in a drink, caffeine is, in fact, an important stimulant for the brain, promoting improved concentration, memory, reaction time and even mood. However, as with all food and drink, the advice is not to overdo it!

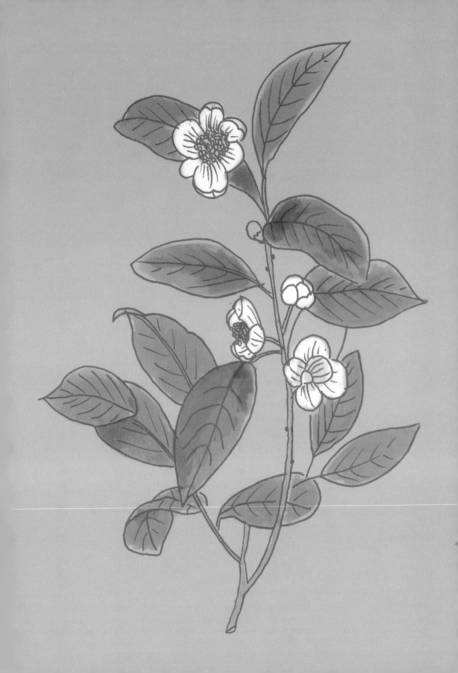

GREEN TEA WITH MINT AND GINGER

Inside: Drink this winter warmer
to soothe a sore throat.

You will need:

1 green tea bag • 4 fresh mint leaves • small piece
fresh ginger

To prepare:

Place the tea bag, mint leaves and a little grated ginger in a
cup. Pour freshly boiled water into the cup and allow the
ingredients to infuse for three minutes. Remove the tea bag
and mint leaves before drinking.

GREEN TEA
STEAM FACIAL TREATMENT

Outside: Combine green tea and lavender for a powerful antibacterial cleanser.

You will need:

2 green tea bags • 4 drops lavender oil

To prepare:

Place the tea bags in a small bowl and cover with freshly boiled water. Allow to infuse for two minutes – it should be cooler but still steaming – then add the lavender oil.

To use:

Lean your face over the bowl with a hand-width distance from your nose to the water. Breathe deeply, allowing the steam to open your pores. Stay in this position as long as is comfortable, then gently splash cool water over your face to refresh and close the pores.

MINT

Mint is a popular herb used the world over for adding a zesty, refreshing flavour to a dish, as a garnish and as a tea. Although there are around fifteen to twenty different types of mint, the most commonly used are spearmint and peppermint. Both grow all year round indoors and thrive outdoors in the summer sunshine.

Mint not only tastes great, it contains small amounts of vitamins A and C, potassium, calcium, phosphorus, magnesium and iron – all important nutrients for healthy skin. It also contains menthol, of course, which works as a decongestant. However, the herb's greatest benefit is the potent antioxidant power it derives from rosmarinic acid, which has proved effective in relieving inflammation and treating a number of other allergy symptoms.

Mint is great to drink as a tea when you have a cold. It relieves sore throats and congestion. It also relieves indigestion and irritable bowel syndrome. When applied to the skin, mint cools and calms redness associated with common skin rashes or insect bites.

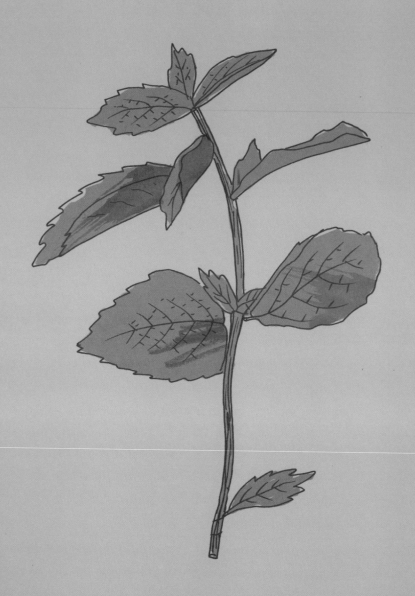

ZINGY MINTY SALAD

Inside: Enjoy this clean-tasting salad for
an antioxidant boost.

You will need:

¼ watermelon • 1 cucumber • 155g feta cheese • 1 bunch of
fresh mint leaves • juice of 1 lime • sea salt • black pepper

To prepare:

Chop the watermelon into dice-sized cubes, remove any seeds
and place in a serving bowl. Trim the cucumber and slice into
thin rounds. Dice the feta and tear or chop the mint leaves,
reserving a few whole leaves for garnish. Add the cucumber,
feta and mint to the serving bowl. Pour over the lime juice and
sprinkle with a pinch of salt and black pepper to taste.

Gently mix all the ingredients to combine thoroughly, then
top with the reserved mint leaves. Serve chilled.

REFRESHING MINT HAIR RINSE

Outside: Refresh and soothe your scalp
while adding extra gloss to your hair.

You will need:

1 peppermint tea bag • 1 teaspoon dried lavender or
chamomile flowers • 125ml freshly boiled water
• 2 tablespoons cider vinegar

To prepare:

Place the tea bag and the dried lavender or chamomile flowers
in a small bowl and cover with the freshly boiled water.
Strain to remove the tea bag and dried flowers, then stir in the
cider vinegar.

To use:

Shampoo and condition your hair as usual then, for the final
rinse, gently massage your scalp and hair with the minty
solution. Dry and style your hair as usual.

BLACK GRAPES

Available all year round, rich, blue-black grapes feature regularly in a healthy Mediterranean diet and are filled with highly beneficial phytonutrients. Their dark colour comes from anthocyanins – anti-inflammatory antioxidant compounds that boost the immune system and keep the skin and body in the best of health.

Black grapes also contain another highly powerful antioxidant, resveratrol, which helps to maintain a healthy circulatory system, ensuring that nourishment reaches skin, hair and nails. These are powerful polyphenols that can help reduce ageing effects in the body – not only in skin but also with memory loss and heart disease.

Great levels of vitamins A, B-complex, C and K, plus health-essential minerals copper, iron, potassium and manganese, make black grapes the perfect superfood dessert choice, especially since they taste sweet and juicy, yet are super low in calories.

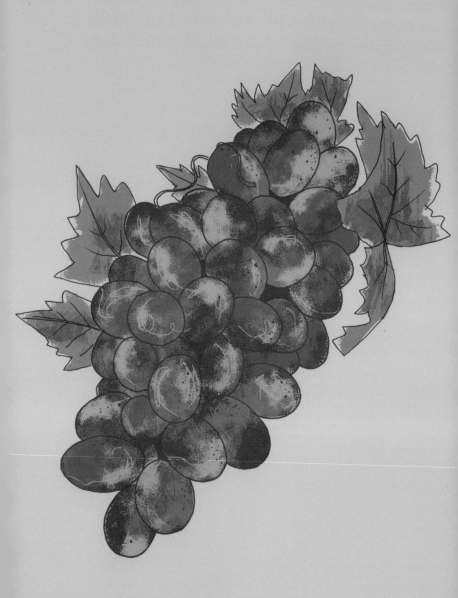

BLACK GRAPE AND RICOTTA SALAD

Inside: Treat yourself to this sweet
anti-ageing dessert.

You will need:

Small bunch of black grapes • 2 tablespoons ricotta • sea salt
• cinnamon • 1 tablespoon toasted hazelnuts • 2 squares
dark chocolate

To prepare:

Wash the black grapes and pat dry. Halve them and place in
a small dish. Place the ricotta in a small bowl, add a pinch of
sea salt and cinnamon, and mix well to combine, then spoon
over the black grape halves. Roughly chop the hazelnuts and
sprinkle them over the ricotta. Grate the dark chocolate over
the top to finish. Serve the salad chilled.

BLACK GRAPE TONER

Outside: Maximize the antioxidant benefits to your skin with this zesty treatment.

You will need:

Small bunch of black grapes • juice of ½ lemon • 4 tablespoons rose water or witch hazel • small clean bottle with lid • cotton ball

To prepare:

Wash the black grapes and place in a blender with the lemon juice and rose water or witch hazel. Blend thoroughly, then strain the juice into a clean bottle to remove the pulp.

To use:

Use a cotton ball to apply the treatment to your skin after cleansing. It will refresh and hydrate. Rose water is best for dryer, more mature skin, while witch hazel is great for younger or more oily skin.

BLUEBERRIES

One of the richest sources of disease-fighting antioxidants,
blueberries are tiny powerhouses of important nutrients
that keep mind and body in the very best of health.

The antioxidant power of blueberries combines with
vitamins A, C, E and K to offer protection from the free-radical
damage that is responsible for premature skin ageing and the
development of some diseases, including cancer and diabetes. It
also improves cell regeneration and strengthens capillaries, resulting
in better skin tone and quality. High levels of anthocyanin – the
compound that gives the blueberry its beautiful skin colour – ensure
clear and healthy eyes. Even brain power is boosted by a daily
handful of these colourful superberries.

This fruit is high in fibre but, unlike many other fruits, low in sugar,
making it the perfect healthy snack. Enjoy fresh, juicy berries
during the summer months or reap the delicious benefits from
frozen berries in winter. They are especially good in a
smoothie or stirred through natural yoghurt.

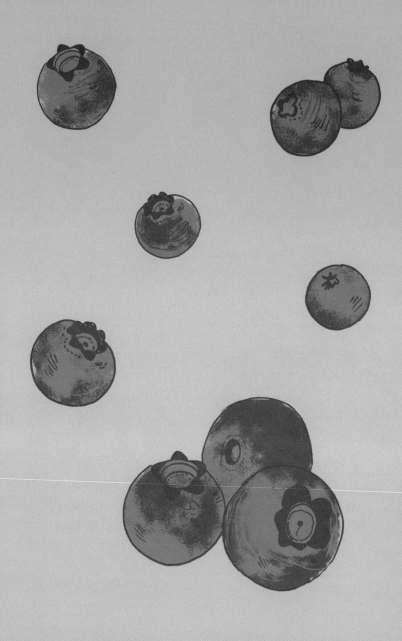

BLUEBERRY AND OAT COOKIES

Inside: Keep your skin looking youthful
with these berry-oaty treats.

You will need:

115g unsalted butter • 185g dark muscovado sugar • 1 egg
• 1 teaspoon vanilla extract • 135g rolled oats • 125g unrefined
flour • ½ teaspoon baking powder • ½ teaspoon salt
• 2 teaspoons cinnamon • 145g blueberries (fresh or frozen)

To prepare:

Preheat the oven to 180 °C/Gas mark 4 and line two baking
trays with greaseproof paper. Cream the butter and sugar
together and add the beaten egg and vanilla extract. Stir
in the oats, flour, baking powder, salt and cinnamon and
combine thoroughly. Gently fold in the blueberries.

Place spoonfuls of the mixture onto the baking trays.
Bake for fifteen minutes until golden, then remove and
place on wire racks to cool.

BLUEBERRY EXFOLIATOR

Outside: Exfoliate, cleanse and condition your skin with this berry-rich blend.

You will need:

35g blueberries • 1 teaspoon sugar • 1 tablespoon olive oil

• 1 tablespoon honey

To prepare:

Blend all the ingredients together until smooth.

To use:

Gently massage the exfoliator in circular strokes across your forehead, down your nose – taking care to avoid the eye area – across your cheeks and around your chin. Rinse off with warm water and pat dry to reveal smooth, glowing skin. This exfoliator is great as a weekly treatment.

CHIA SEEDS

The power of this nutrient-packed, energy-boosting superseed was recognized by the ancient Aztecs and Mayans. The word 'chia' meant 'strength' to the Mayans and they would use the seeds both as a medicine and as an everyday food.

Just one tablespoon of chia seeds, which are also gluten-free, contains a highly effective mix of vital vitamins and minerals, oils, protein and fibre, to keep the body and brain in peak condition. With high levels of antioxidants and essential fatty acids – predominantly omega-3 – chia seeds help ensure skin, hair and nails are well nourished. Impressive levels of protein offer a good balance of essential amino acids for healthy body function and the high fibre content helps to regulate blood sugar levels and keep the digestive system running well.

Good levels of calcium, manganese, magnesium, phosphorus, zinc, potassium and B-complex vitamins simply add to this tiny seed's power as the ultimate beauty weapon! Grown all year round in Mexico, chia seeds can last up to two years without losing their nutritional effectiveness – a great indication of their antioxidant power!

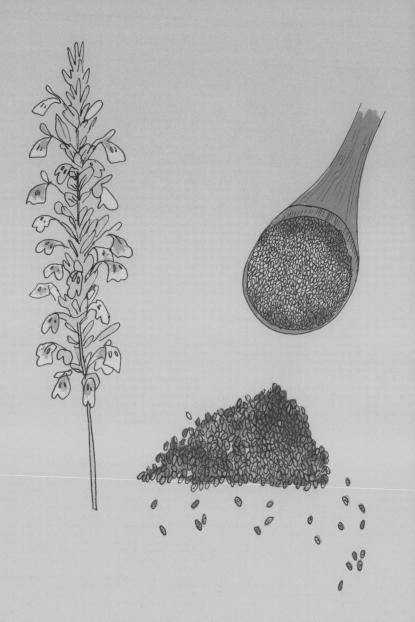

CHIA BREAKFAST SMOOTHIE

Inside: Give yourself a protein boost with this rich breakfast smoothie.

You will need:

1 ripe banana • 1 tablespoon chia seeds • 1 tablespoon organic peanut butter • 1 teaspoon raw honey • 250ml whole milk • ground cinnamon

To prepare:

Chop the banana and place in a blender with the chia seeds, peanut butter, honey and milk. Blend until rich and creamy and pour into a serving glass.

Sprinkle with cinnamon for a potassium-, calcium- and protein-rich breakfast that will give you all the energy you need for a busy morning.

CHIA SKIN AND LIP OIL

Outside: Use this great winter treatment to
hydrate even the driest lips and skin.

You will need:

1 tablespoon chia seeds • 250ml spring water • 1 teaspoon
coconut oil

To prepare:

Place the chia seeds in a small glass bowl, cover with spring
water, and leave to soak overnight. The seeds will absorb
the water and form a gel-like consistency. Add the coconut oil
and mix thoroughly.

To use:

Spread the treatment over your face and lips. Leave on for
thirty minutes to moisturize. Your skin will glow with
radiance and your lips will be plump and smooth.

DATES

This superfood of the desert can be eaten fresh when in season –
during autumn – or all year round in its dried form. Dates are grown
in the dry, arid conditions of Egypt and the Middle East and have a
concentration of important vitamins and minerals. So much so,
that many people believe that it is possible to survive for days in
the desert with just water to drink and dates to eat.

A rich source of antioxidants, these sweet palm fruits are also high
in calcium, iron, potassium, phosphorus, manganese, magnesium and
copper, all of which contribute to strong muscle development as well as
healthy skin and hair. A high dietary fibre content helps regulate the
digestive system, while promoting good bacteria in the intestines – and
good digestion means improved absorption of nutrients from all
foods. All in all, dates make a perfect, satisfying snack that
leaves you glowing with health inside and out.

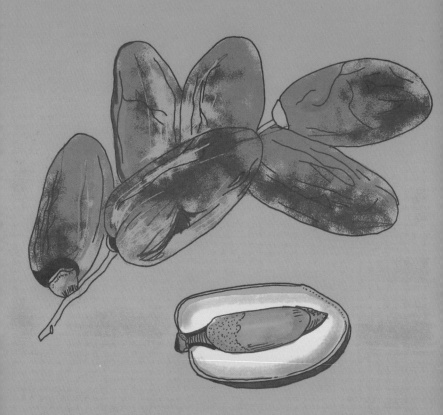

DATE AND BEETROOT BLISS BALLS

Inside: Boost your muscle development with these mineral-rich delights.

You will need:

250g dried dates • 140g almonds • 85g dried, shredded coconut • 175g finely grated beetroot • 1 tablespoon coconut oil • 1 teaspoon fresh ginger, finely chopped (optional) • juice of ½ lemon

To prepare:

Remove the pits from the dates and place all the ingredients – except the lemon juice – in a food processor. Blend until the ingredients are finely processed and you have a soft, dough-like paste – if it's too solid add a little lemon juice.

Taking a little of the mixture at a time, roll it in your hands to form bite-sized balls. Place them on a baking tray and refrigerate for fifteen minutes before eating.

DATE, YOGHURT AND HONEY FACE MASK

Outside: Cleanse and nourish your face for a radiant and youthful complexion.

You will need:

4 dried dates • 1 cup warm water • 1 tablespoon thick yoghurt
• 1 teaspoon clear honey

To prepare:

Remove the pits from the dates and soak in warm water for one hour. Drain, and place in a blender along with the yoghurt and honey. Blend together until smooth.

To use:

Gently massage the mask onto your face – right up to the eyes and down the neck. Leave for fifteen minutes, before rinsing off with warm water to reveal softer, refreshed and healthier looking skin.

OLIVES

Juicy green or rich black olives have long been considered a health promoting food throughout the Mediterranean. Ripe and ready for harvest during the summer months, they are rich in antioxidants, important minerals and vitamins, good omega-6 and omega-3 oils and phytosterols, which are great for helping reduce cholesterol and keeping your heart healthy. Rich in skin-loving vitamin E and carotenoids, olives also help protect against inflammation and keep the nervous system healthy.

Olives contain good quantities of calcium, manganese, iron, copper and zinc, as well as essential B-complex vitamins, all of which contribute to smooth, supple skin and shiny hair. Cold-pressed, virgin olive oil is the best to use in salad dressings: not only does this have optimum nutritional value, it also has the best taste!

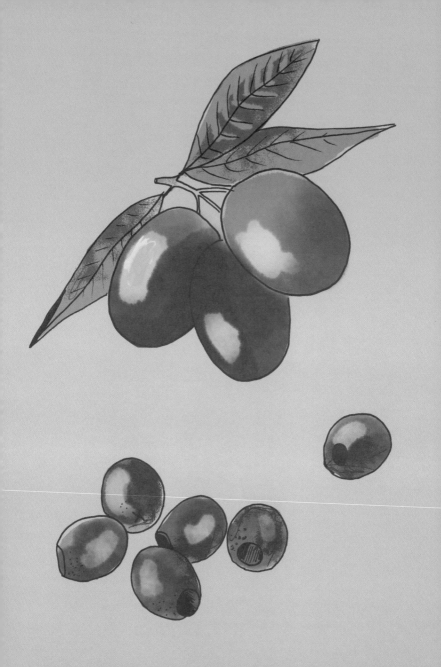

MARINATED OLIVES WITH FETA

Inside: Boost your heart health with
this phytosterol-rich dish.

You will need:

75g black pitted olives • 200g feta cheese • sprig of
rosemary • juice of ½ lemon • 1 tablespoon olive oil • sea salt
• black pepper

To prepare:

Chop the olives, dice the feta and place both in a small serving
bowl. Chop the rosemary leaves and add to the bowl along
with the lemon juice and the olive oil. Dust with sea salt and
black pepper and leave the flavours to infuse for thirty
minutes. Serve on crackers or toasted sourdough.

OLIVE OIL HAIR TREATMENT

Outside: Apply this deep-reaching, vitamin E-rich
oil for softer, glossier hair.

You will need:

1 egg yolk • 2 tablespoons olive oil • 1 teaspoon lemon juice

To prepare:

Beat the egg yolk in a small bowl then add the olive oil and
lemon juice and combine thoroughly.

To use:

Massage the mixture into dry hair, taking care to include
the ends. Leave for fifteen minutes, then rinse away in
warm water and shampoo and condition as usual. The result?
Shiny, supersoft hair.

SEAWEED

There are many types of edible seaweed available – including kelp, spirulina and red and brown algae. Although these seaweeds are popular and available as dried powders for mixing into smoothies or sprinkling over salads and soups, the most easily available seaweed is nori, which can be bought dried and in sheets.

Seaweed is rich in chlorophyll, a great natural detoxifier and alkalizer of the blood. It is also a welcome source of vitamin K, which is important for healthy blood formation. Seaweed's high iodine content ensures optimum functioning of the thyroid gland, which produces the essential hormones for all the body's cells in addition to regulating the metabolism. Other valuable nutrients include vitamins A and B12, omega-3 essential fatty acids and a high level of calcium, all of which contribute to healthy skin, hair and nails.

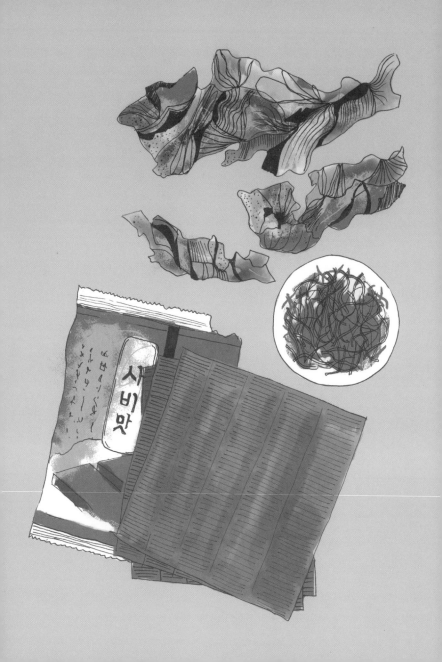

NORI WRAPS

Inside: Make these chlorophyll-rich wraps
for a cleansing, alkalizing boost.

You will need:

½ ripe avocado • juice of ½ lemon • sea salt • black pepper
• 1 carrot • 3 dried nori sheets • chilli flakes • 3 cooked
asparagus spears • 1 handful spinach leaves

To prepare:

Mash the avocado with the lemon juice and add salt and
pepper to taste. Peel the carrot and cut into thin sticks. Lay
out the nori sheets, spread each with avocado and sprinkle
with chilli flakes.

Layer the carrot sticks, asparagus spears and spinach leaves
along one edge of each nori sheet, then roll to form the wrap.
Serve immediately.

SEAWEED FACE MASK

Outside: Try this powerful hydration boost for a youthful complexion.

You will need:

2 nori sheets • 1 cup freshly boiled spring water

To prepare:

This is the simplest of all homemade beauty treatments! Allow the boiled water to cool. While still warm, pour the water over the nori sheets and leave until softened.

To use:

Break small sections off the nori sheet and apply all over your face, pressing into your skin and avoiding the eye area. Close your eyes and relax for twenty minutes. Remove the seaweed using a tissue and rinse your skin in warm water. Pat dry to reveal soft and glowing skin.

RECIPE FINDER

RECIPES

BEAUTY TREATMENTS

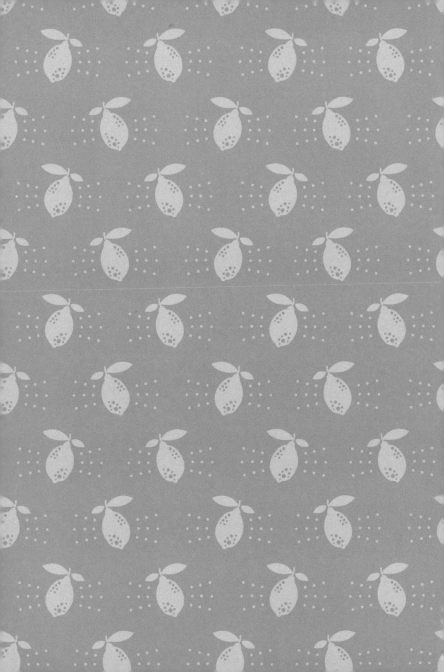